BEDTIME,
the Ultimate
BATTLE

BEDTIME,
the Ultimate
BATTLE

A Parent's Sleep Guide for Infants and Toddlers

MELISSA GUIDA-RICHARDS

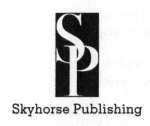

Skyhorse Publishing

Skyhorse Publishing books may be purchased in bulk at special discounts for sales promotion, corporate gifts, fund-raising, or educational purposes. Special editions can also be created to specifications. For details, contact the Special Sales Department, Skyhorse Publishing, 307 West 36th Street, 11th Floor, New York, NY 10018 or info@skyhorsepublishing.com.

Skyhorse® and Skyhorse Publishing® are registered trademarks of Skyhorse Publishing, Inc.®, a Delaware corporation.

Visit our website at www.skyhorsepublishing.com.

10 9 8 7 6 5 4 3 2 1

Library of Congress Cataloging-in-Publication Data is available on file.

Cover design by Laura Klynstra
Cover photo credit Getty Images

Print ISBN: 978-1-5107-4518-6
Ebook ISBN: 978-1-5107-4519-3

Printed in the United States of America

For my boys, Carlito and Killian.

For my boys. Go make a difference.

CONTENTS

PRIMING FOR BATTLE

They told you it would happen. You laughed, smiled, and agreed. But, deep down inside, you didn't believe it would be *that* bad. You're almost there. It's okay. I got you. I will help you through this. It's okay, I'm here now.

But I need you to do one thing first:

Accept the fact that you will *never* get enough sleep.

I know, I know.

It's hard, and you're probably thinking, *No, I can't. I need sleep. My baby needs sleep. We will both eventually sleep through the night.* Well, stranger, you got me there. Yes, you both will sleep through the night. I can confidently say every baby will sleep through the night at some point, but what I don't think you know is that even if you get eight hours of sweet, sweet shut-eye every night, it will *never* be enough. Your baby will wake up like a real-life mini version of you as the energizer bunny, and then you will rub your eyes, hoping that once you've washed your face and showered, you'll feel better. After all, you got enough sleep, right? You slept eight hours!

The reality is . . . it's *never* enough. And once you accept that, you're ready to try anything that will get you *just enough* sleep to function.

It's okay. You can be mad at me. Throw this book on the floor, and yell, cry, and try the swaddle for the thousandth time. I'll be here when you're ready.

Feel free to rip this blank page out if you want.
Or punch a pillow.
I know sleep deprivation can cause anger issues.

Oh, hey! You came back.

I'm truly and deeply sorry that this is happening to you. I understand. Really, I do. For about three years I've been a premium member of Parents on the Struggle Bus. This is why I'm writing this. Parents need to stick together and keep each other from losing it after the millionth-and-one-night of not enough sleep.

I got you.

I'm just a parent like you, who has spent countless hours on the Internet Googling how to get my kid to fall asleep. I'm just a normal-ish millennial mama, who is trying to survive two toddlers who act more like monkeys most days. But I think I found a system that works and I felt the need to share it with my friends, family, and now you. Since we are on this journey together, facing the Bedtime Battle, I thought I would do my best to help my fellow parents and guardians. We need to stick together!

After countless late nights breastfeeding each baby, and rocking, swaddling, and singing, I thought that there ought to be a guide out there that was easy for a sleep-deprived parent to follow. In the twenty-first century, we are often on the go, and I know I didn't have the time or energy to devote myself to one method, especially when my children would change their preferences on a nightly basis sometimes.

This book will be your answer to a better night's sleep. Sometimes, if you're lucky, a full night of sleep. Or, often just a long enough stretch of unconsciousness that you manage to feed your baby the mashed peas and not the dog food.

In this book, you will find many useful tips that I will personally swear by, and you will find some that may seem ridiculous but that the Internet swears by. Either way, check with your doctor first.

Each section correlates with a phase of sleep that I've personally experienced as a parent battling bedtime. For example, my kids were really into movement as a means of getting them to sleep, and if your babies are the same, you may want to check out Chapter Six: Motion of the Ocean. When they were having some bodily changes like a tummy ache from gas, or reflux, I created Biological Warfare. Chapter 5: Leveling Up, is dedicated to the leaps that you may have heard about that come with each new stage in development as your baby learns a new skill. It did a wonder on our sleep situation at home, and I knew I had to create a section to help my fellow parents out, as well.

I'm not a magician, and my tips will not be the cure to your sleep situation, but they can help. This guide is something I wished I had had when I was a lonely mom, with postpartum, struggling to make it through to the next day on no sleep. The Internet saved me, with tips and tricks, but I had to dig and read over articles with the same tips over and over before finding something that worked for my family. This is my gift to every parent, especially those without a support system. I know what it's like living far away from family, with no babysitter, while your husband works crazy hours. I know what it's like being pregnant and still needing to wake up with a baby.

So, with all of my heart, I wish you the best of luck on your parenting journey. I hope that *Bedtime, The Ultimate Battle*, makes it a little easier in your house every night. Good luck, sweet dreams, and if you have any questions, feel free to reach out to me via my website Guida-Richards.com.

CHAPTER ONE
SAFETY FIRST

I know you're in a rush, but **do not** skip this chapter. I'll make this quick and painless. This chapter is important for everyone with a baby. It is especially useful, if you are a newbie and have never held more than a Baby Alive or an American Girl Doll, but it is also a great reminder for all caregivers because it focuses on safety!

Most of these tips are infant-related, but it is still wise to use general caution with your older children, as well. Just because your baby can roll over does not mean a mountain of stuffed animals is now safe. Please use common sense and ask your doctor if you have any specific questions about what is right for your child.

1. Consult your pediatrician! There are weird things out there, silly things, and even some danger-ous ones. This book contains dozens of tips that are useful, but depending on your baby's health, your health, and the environment you live in, they may not all be safe for your family. And that's okay! You *will* find what works for your family.

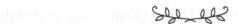

2. Keep that baby flatter than a pancake. Experts have discovered that a firm, flat surface is by far the safest of options for your baby to sleep on. Save the Tempur-Pedic bed for later and use the money you would spend on a fancy, fluffy bed on a nice tall cup of coffee instead.

3. My friends, stop buying bumpers, toys, and all sorts of (let's be honest) junk that your baby doesn't care about and putting it in their crib. It's not safe. Don't you dare *oh, well I had it when I was a baby and I'm fine* me. 'Cause guess what? A bunch of babies got hurt when you were a baby, too. If you know better, do better.

3

4. This one is easy! **Make sure your baby is wearing fitted clothing.** Save the frills, bear suits, and costumes for when baby *and you* are awake. Trust me, it's more fun that way because you can't post to social media when you're asleep. Think of all the likes you'll get to enjoy during the four o'clock morning feed.

5. Slightly repetitive, but it's necessary to remind you: **Don't use special sleep products in the crib.** No pool noodles, wedges, lava lamps, or thingamajigs. Keep it simple! Plus, look at it this way: it's one fewer thing to remember to find when you're sleep deprived.

CHAPTER TWO
THE NEWBORN NEMESIS

You thought your baby was cute, innocent, and perfect. But even perfect babies have difficulties falling asleep. Even though it can be the hardest stage, and feels like it lasts forever, it's just a small fraction of your life. So, without further ado, here are the best tips for newborn sleep.

6. Use white noise. Fun fact—a mother's womb is loud. The beating of the mother's heart, the musical sounds of digestion, and the vibrating echo of the outside world create a symphony of sounds your baby is familiar with and, frankly, dependent on. So, do yourself a favor and buy a white noise machine. Preferably one with lots of options (like waves, heartbeat, and static).

7. Allow a pacifier. Binky, booboo, dumdum, nipple, baba, or whatever you like to call it. One thing is certain—babies love suckling. It's comforting and can often help soothe them to sleep, and whether the mother breastfeeds or not does not change this instinct. However, you need to know that not all pacifiers are worthy in the eyes of your beloved baby. You've never seen a truly fickle person until you've seen a baby reject a dozen different types of pacifiers.

Which means don't stock up on cute Wubbanubs in case your baby decides they hate them, otherwise you'll be wasting money. Buy a couple different kinds first, and keep trying, just like a lovesick teenager. Eventually, if you are persistent, even the most stubborn babies will learn to take one.

8. Become a swaddling expert. The nurses made it look so easy in the hospital. I will break it down for ya. First put that sweet little angel on the floor somewhere safe. Next, grab your weapon of choice: the swaddle. It doesn't matter what color or design, but a cute little bunny rabbit may make you more optimistic (personally, I prefer penguins).

Step 1: Lay the swaddle on the floor and fold one corner a quarter of the way down.

Step 2: Place your baby with his head above the part you folded down (baby will be diagonal across the blanket).

Step 3: Pull the left corner tightly across his body and tuck it underneath.

Step 4: Gently pull the bottom corner up so it covers his legs and arm. Tuck that end underneath their shoulder, and there should be enough room for your baby's legs to move.

Step 5: Pull the remaining corner tight across his body while making sure his arm is straight and tuck it snugly underneath.

Step 6: Admire your handiwork.

If your swaddle looks anything like the nurse's swaddle job in the hospital, you are the real MVP. If you suck at swaddling, make your partner try. Then, if they can't figure it out, I give you permission to buy easy Velcro swaddles. 10/10 would recommend.

9. Consider supplementing with formula. As a sleep-deprived parent, you're desperate. You may have committed to breastfeeding at first. Then it was a struggle waking up every few hours to nurse that cute, shrieking baby. It's now a couple days or weeks in, and the reality of the situation sinks in: you are the only person with lactating breasts who can feed your child, and now you start to wonder . . .

Are the rumors true? Do formula-fed babies sleep through the night? Am I not making enough milk? My partner should be helping!

Short answer: they will probably sleep in longer spurts than breastfed babies.

Long answer: Well, here's the deal. *Some* formula-fed babies sleep through the night. And *some* don't. Formula takes longer for the baby's body to digest, so even if they don't sleep all night long, they will likely sleep longer than a breastfed baby.

Breast milk contains the perfect amount of nutrients for the baby and therefore it digests super quickly. So, is it worth a shot? Sure! Am I promising you a full night's rest? Not at all!

10. Continue skin to skin: Babies love the smell of their mothers. They have just spent nine months in your womb, and every time they lay on their mom's chest, endorphins are released, which is relaxing for both Mom and baby. So, for the first couple of weeks, it's normal for the baby to need to sleep on Mom.

If you're nervous about co-sleeping, try to switch sleep shifts with your partner so they can keep an eye on the baby. My husband and I would take turns holding the baby while the other one was awake for the first few weeks of his life because we were worried about dropping him while asleep.

11. Swing, baby, swing! In the womb, babies are almost constantly being rocked by the motions of their mama. Try out that baby swing that you received at your baby shower from your Great-Aunt Susie. It just might be your lifesaver.

My first baby refused to sleep unless he was constantly rocked, and since my hubby had to work from Day 1, we ended up relying on the baby swing for some sanity. Ours was a fancy one that played a dozen different sounds and musical tones. It was definitely worth every penny. Always transfer your baby out and into a safe sleeping space, and as always, never leave them unsupervised.

12. Take a trip to Boob Town. If you're breastfeeding, utilize your powers when you can. Baby's hungry? Give 'em the boob. Baby is gassy? Boob. Baby needs a nap? You got it, boob time!

Breast milk is truly magical. It adjusts to the baby's needs throughout the day. At night, your milk will contain hormones that will help baby sleep. Don't worry about creating a habit and making baby dependent on the boob for sleep right now. In the first couple of weeks, it's solely about survival. They won't become dependent until they're a little older, and you can wean them off it then.

13. Carpe Diem! Live life to the fullest and enjoy every second that you can. Your baby will never be little again. This time is magical as well as challenging, and you may be learning that your expectations of motherhood or fatherhood were completely off base. You may be struggling and barely getting by, or you may be rocking the sh*t out of this parenting thing. Either way, it's important to remember that you are only human and to try to find the best in the situation.

Baby has barely slept a wink off of you? You've ordered takeout every day for the past three weeks? Your partner is stuck sleeping on the couch? Baby weight not coming off?

Try and rephrase the situation.

Baby loves you so much and they find comfort in simply touching you. You fed yourself and your family! Your partner is willing to sacrifice his comfort for his family's best interests. You're giving your body a break from dieting to concentrate on the baby you created the past nine months. That all sounds, and feels, a lot better, right?

WHAT WORKED FOR YOU?

Tip	Success	Fail
Use white noise	☐	☐
Allow a pacifier	☐	☐
Becoming a swaddling expert	☐	☐
Supplement with formula	☐	☐
Continue skin to skin	☐	☐
Swing, baby, swing!	☐	☐
Take a trip to Boob Town	☐	☐
Carpe Diem!	☐	☐

WHAT WORKED FOR YOU?

CHAPTER THREE
THE CLASSICS

Little Women, Moby Dick, Pride and Prejudice, The Godfather, Casablanca, and *The Wizard of Oz* all have one thing in common. They are The Classics. Whether you personally like them or not, you can recognize that they contain key plot elements that make them special. They may not work for everyone, every time, but once you find the one that you love, it will never let you down.

These are the classic bedtime moves that every parent needs to have in their arsenal. Once you know your baby's chosen one, use that for all its worth. The thing about babies is that they're fickler than adults, so it's best to find a couple techniques they love so you can alternate on an especially difficult night.

14. Bath time! My first baby loved baths from the start, and my youngest sounded like he was being waterboarded the entire time. May the odds be ever in your favor, and if your child is not the next Michael Phelps, try taking a bath with them.

You can also set the mood with some sleepy-time baby bath wash that smells like lavender. Make sure to keep your movements slow and gentle and add some lullaby music in the background. If your laundry area is nearby or if your partner is around to help you out, stick a towel in the dryer for a few minutes to help transition your baby out and into some snug pajamas as you go about the rest of your routine.

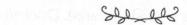

15. Be a mommy masseuse. Stress. Everybody experiences it. Even that tiny little newborn cooing softly in your arms. New places, lights, smells, and gas can stress out their little systems quicker than you can think. It can be extremely beneficial to give your angel a gentle massage before bed. Pick up your favorite lotion and gently rub it into their skin. Add a soft lullaby in the background and lower the lights to set the mood for sleep.

I know that I pass out every time I get a massage, therefore it may be a great idea to try and create that feeling of relaxation with your baby to ease them into an easier bedtime routine.

16. Nightly story time. It's never too early to begin reading to your child. Starting a nightly ritual of a bedtime story is perfect for creating a routine that helps wind down your little cherub for the night. Try out simple black-and-white board books, describe scenes out loud in a soft voice, and you may find your sweetie drifting off to the land of sleep sooner than you expected.

Why? Babies love hearing their parents' voices since they recognize them from their time in the womb. As you get into the routine of reading and snuggling your baby for the night, it will help ease you both into winding down for bed. As your child gets older, she will pay more attention to the images that will help stimulate her brain and give her something to focus on as she drifts off. The distraction may be just the thing you need to help baby sleep.

It always seems like when you want your child to drift off, they won't, so try going into bedtime with a different mentality. If they know that it's story time, and not yet bedtime, they may not fight as hard.

17. Give in to dream-feeding. This can be done with a boob or a bottle. Yay, options!

As we parents know, it is vital to feed our tiny humans before they drift off to lala land. But, after a longggg day of changing diapers, rocking, and dealing with a shrieking banshee, you are probably not going to sleep right away. You're going to cash in on some quality adult time drinking wine, binging Netflix, or actually talking to your spouse. Before you know it, it's pushing eleven at night and you're pulling up the covers in your comfortable bed when you hear it.

Okay, maybe it's not real. You're just imagining the baby cry.

But then it grows louder and louder until you know your baby is going to bust a lung, so you hurry up, grab your phone and a bottle (or your boobs, feeling for which one is fuller), and you run to your tiny human.

Now, I'm gonna tell you how to avoid this whole situation.

If your baby wakes up two or three hours after bedtime, plan to sneak into their room for a little midnight snack before you head to bed. If you're breastfeeding, I recommend pumping a bottle so you don't have to pick up the little nugget, and/or send your partner into the room to dream-feed.

Babies can nurse in their sleep, so as long as formula or breastmilk is the only thing in the bottle, you may find your angel sleeping for a longer stretch. As always, consult your doctor before changing any feeds. Simply prepare a small bottle and feed it to them right before they would usually wake up for a feeding. You'll be surprised at how this does the trick!

18. Patty cake, patty cake! To be honest, I'm not really sure why this works. The prevalent theory is that it replicates the mother's heartbeat and is therefore familiar and soothing. All I know is that most babies *love* it. So many times, I've stood over my son's crib patting his back or his bum and found that he fell asleep faster than it took me to change his poopy diaper. The type of pressure depends on the baby, so try switching things up with soft or hard pats, slow or fast, to find the settings that lull your little cherub into slumber.

19. Blackout. The night is dark and full of . . . tired parents trying to get their kids to fall asleep. Now, this may seem obvious, but in case you are too exhausted to realize this, I'll say it here: make sure your baby's room is dark AF. This means blackout curtains, no night-lights, and definitely do not shine your phone light on them to make sure they are breathing fifty times a night.

Same goes for naps. Keep screens away for at least an hour before they need to sleep, and make sure they're getting their vitamin D from the sun during the day to adjust their sleep schedules so they do not continue to be night owls.

20. Naptime is important. Again I say: *Naptime is important.* I will cherish naptime until it goes away. For your little tyke to get into a great sleep routine at night, they will need to take one to three *quality* naps before bedtime. And yes, oh sleepy one, I said *quality.* Because quality over quantity counts with naps. You may read a thousand baby books that say your baby needs four forty-minute naps per minute of age, or month of the year, or the same number of naps as the number of feet of the animal on the Chinese Calendar year that your baby was born on. But the frustrating truth is that every single baby is different, and some babies will fight you on that every single day.

21. Upgrade your diapers. Pee your pants. I dare you. You won't. Okay, just imagine you spilled coffee on yourself again, and now you're going to sleep with about a full cup's worth on your soft PJs. Now, try to sleep in those clothes. Doesn't sound so cozy, right? No! Do yourself and your baby a favor and find the optimal diaper situation, whether that means extra cloth inserts or some heavy-duty super-soaker Nimbus 2000s. Upgrade your beloved's sweet tush situation if they are leaking or have started waking up early for some unknown reason. It may just be that their diapers are getting fuller sooner than usual and they are still too tiny to tell you with more than just screeching Chewbacca noises. To win this battle, try a size up for nighttime.

22. Find your child's favorite lullaby. Now, this one may sound easy and obvious. You have the tried-and-true ones like "Go to Sleep," "Rockabye Baby," and my favorite one from The Cheetah Girls, "A La Nanita." Or, you can switch things up like my husband showed me and try some, shall I say, alternative music choices. Our first-born son loved screamo and our youngest adored musicals. It may be weird at first, and you may need some ear plugs until your child drifts off into a peaceful slumber. You may even find that he needs the song played all night long and you cannot get a second's worth of peace because you're stuck listening to it over the baby monitor even when it's on the lowest setting. But, hey, at least your baby is sleeping, right?

23. Pre-game. Before taking care of your little love, you need to pre-game. Get yourself ready for the big game before kickoff. Take a minute for yourself to go use the restroom, to grab your phone, or your water bottle—whatever it is that you need to do before you are trapped under a ticking timebomb. Do you crochet? Is your phone charger handy? Do you have midnight snacks within arm's reach in the nursery? And most importantly, do you have diaper supplies fully stocked and food for the baby?

WHAT WORKED FOR YOU?

Tip	Success	Fail
Bath time	☐	☐
Mommy masseuse	☐	☐
Story time	☐	☐
Dream-feeding	☐	☐
Patty cake!	☐	☐
Blackout	☐	☐
Naptime	☐	☐
Diaper upgrade	☐	☐
Favorite lullaby	☐	☐
Pre-game	☐	☐

CHAPTER FOUR
CHEAT CODES

There are no true "hacks" to getting a baby to sleep, but there sure are different ones the Internet claims you can try. After all, if they're safe and you're going to be up anyway, you may as well entertain yourself trying. I've included some of these funky tips because tired parents need a laugh, and in the process, you may find a weird thing that relaxes your babe. The key to good sleep is a stress-free environment, and by having a little fun, you can make the battle a little easier.

24. Become Dr. Phil. When I was studying to get my degree in psychology, we learned about observing people's behavior in order to conduct studies. One of the best things I ever did for our family was become my baby's personal Dr. Phil. I took note of when he needed his naps most, when he wanted to breastfeed versus eat solids, and whether he did better with an

>>

earlier bedtime versus a later one. Basically, I took note of anything and everything trying to crack the code.

Eventually, I figured out a system that worked for my family. Most people need an early bedtime, but for a good couple of months, my firstborn would sleep through the night only if he went to bed at 10 p.m. and not a minute earlier after breastfeeding to sleep, and my husband had to be the one to lay him in his crib. After that, I couldn't get within a five-foot radius of his room or he'd wake up. Babies are like complicated Rubik's cubes, and once you crack the code, the puzzle changes and you have to Dr. Phil them all over again.

25. Record a voice memo. When babies are in the womb, they are constantly bombarded with noises from the outside world, and then all of a sudden, they are earth-side and are alone in a quiet room when it's time to sleep. That can be more than just a little scary for a newborn or even an infant. So, what can you do? Take an old smartphone and download a voice memo app, and then pick up a book and record yourself talking for at least an hour. Now you can play it for your baby until they fall into a deeper sleep.

26. Try the tissue trick. If you have the Internet, I'm pretty sure you've seen the adorable video of the baby falling asleep after having a tissue gently drifting over his face for about a minute. Now, if you live under a rock, go Google it. I'll wait. I tried it, and believe it or not, it works … for about a minute or two. But my firstborn was a Velcro baby who needed to be attached to me 24/7, so it wasn't a real solution. I didn't bother trying with my second because he slept so well, so you'll have to let me know how that goes long term.

27. Discover alternative white noises. White noise is a classic baby sleep aid and always will be. It will come to your aid time and time again. Some babies like fans, some like music boxes, and some like the sound of the ocean played on a fancy white noise machine that cost a hundred bucks from the baby shower. Keep trying different weird sounds until one clicks. Hopefully, it's something that won't make you want to stab your ears every night over the baby's crib. My husband is into screamo and would play it often to our boys. I hope your solution is a little easier on your ears.

28. Create a Winter Wonderland. To my fellow Americans, it may seem taboo, but in other countries such as Norway and Scandinavia, babies can actually nap outside in the cold. Now, before you get your panties in a twist, take a deep breath. Of course, the infants are dressed extra snug in appropriate jackets and blankets, but people have actually found that babies nap better in colder climates, and it is commonplace to find babies napping in their strollers outside cafes as parents grab a coffee or snack. So, you may want to consider keeping the nursery a degree or two colder than you would normally and putting your baby in a cozy sleeper if they're having trouble sleeping at night.

29. The nose knows. Kids have a sixth sense, especially little babies. Did you know that a newborn can pick the blanket their mother was holding out of a line-up, by just the way it smells? You can use this trick to your advantage by wearing their bedsheets around for an hour or so before putting them to bed. I used to shove the sheet in my bra, because I was breastfeeding and the closer it was to my milk stash, the easier my baby was tricked. This battle will probably be easier for Mom to win because of basic biology, but I'm sure if Dad is the primary caregiver it can be pretty effective, too.

30. Play Tug of War. Desperate times call for desperate measures. If all else fails, you may want to follow one Internet father's lead: He placed his baby on a blanket in his living room and gently pulled her around until she fell asleep. Is this unconventional? Yes. Effective? Maybe. If you're desperate enough and your baby isn't the wiggly type, you might as well give it a try. At the very least, it will be amusing for the both of you, and at this point of sleep deprivation, you both need a laugh.

31. Plan to party hard! Take a hint from the stars and *get lit*! During the day, that is. Some kids have a hard time sleeping at night because they're still working out the kinks in their sleep schedules. One of the easiest ways to help them learn how to transition from each sleep cycle is to wear them out during the day. Take them to the park, the zoo, the store, or whatever you need to do to make them tired . . . even if it's letting them watch a little more television than they usually do. Until they are on a good sleep schedule, it's okay to operate in survival mode.

WHAT WORKED FOR YOU?

Tip	Success	Fail
Become Dr. Phil	☐	☐
Voice memo	☐	☐
Tissue trick	☐	☐
Alternative white noise	☐	☐
Winter Wonderland	☐	☐
Nose knows	☐	☐
Tug-of-War	☐	☐
Party hard!	☐	☐

CHAPTER FIVE
LEVELING UP

With each new stage in development, your baby may struggle with falling to sleep. Babies grow so fast that their new skills can be overwhelming and can lead to overstimulation, which . . . well, you know where this is gonna go. Each new skill like vocalization, sitting up, walking, and then talking can make the world seem like an even bigger and more interesting place than it was.

Now, if you were a baby, wouldn't you feel like you were missing out on things if you went to bed? This is why it's important to adapt and change with your child so *you* don't get stuck in the land of sleep deprivation. Here are some tips to help you survive each new challenge, or as some would call them, sleep regressions.

32. Squat, baby, squat! This one is pretty hard on your glutes. You can strap your baby in a carrier if you want, or hold them securely against your chest as you squat over and over . . . and over, until your baby relaxes. This tip is great, because you can't fall asleep while moving around, and the bouncing will give you some exercise that might help you sleep easier, as well. Now, you may want to stretch beforehand because your legs may eventually cramp. The problem with this little handy maneuver is that your little angel may love it so much they may not want you to ever stop.

33. Always have backup. Your child has a favorite binky? Stock up. Favorite diaper? Blankie or lovey? Definitely stock up. Favorite bedtime bubble bath and lotion? You better stock up on that special lavender scent. If you find something that works, and it seems like it's going to go out of stock or it's something that you will probably lose, make sure you have extras. You will thank me later. Bonus points if you tell dear old Grandma and Grandpa to have one or two of their favorite giraffe teethers at their house, so you have a spare. You can always write a review or call the company reviewing their product in hopes for a sweet little coupon to take the edge off the pain of your wallet burning.

34. Become a Dancing Queen. When in doubt, dance it out! Seriously. Dance to anything. Happy, sad, romantic, hard rock. Babies love to be rocked and rolled all night long, and let's be honest, what's better than a party with Mommy and Daddy at two in the morning? Remember that for nine months, little Johnny was being rocked to sleep in the womb as Mom walked around, cooked, cleaned, and hiked. Nights were when he partied as you lay snuggled in bed, so it's important to try to replicate similar patterns now that he is earth-side.

35. Avoid eye contact. This is pretty much an unspoken rule, and I'm gonna break it down for you, because I like you. After all, you're reading my book. Babies can sense when you're trying to put them to bed, and the second your eyes meet their hooded little peepers, they will pop open faster than you can say, "Sandman!" Without a doubt, one of you will be crying in the next few minutes.

To combat this, try one of the previous tips, and for the love of all the hopes and dreams in the world, do not look your baby in the eyes to check if she's sleeping. Strategically glance in her general direction, cautiously pull up selfie mode on your phone, or just listen for the cute baby snores. Whatever you do, *don't* look her in the eyes.

36. Bring the heat(ing pad). This is a magic trick I thought would never work, but it does for some babies. Others, *cough*, like my second child, aren't phased, but for the chosen ones, it's a game changer. Take a heating pad and lay it on the baby's crib mattress or play yard for a few minutes, until the surface is warm. Check the area to be sure it isn't too hot, and then gently place your baby on their bed after you rock/sing/dance them to sleep. If you don't have an electric heating pad, you can make a heating pad out of an old sock and rice and warm it up in the microwave in thirty-second increments.

37. Consider a Heartbeat Bear. Okay, so they (various companies, you can find them online with a quick search) make this stuffed animal that's kind of creepy but useful as hell. It has a heartbeat to trick your baby into thinking they are co-sleeping with their mom. Pros, it's a cute stuffed animal your baby can play with and love. Cons, you need to consider SIDS and safe sleeping practices. Personally, I didn't use it, but I know tons of moms who swear by this adorable, only mildly terrifying stuffed animal.

38. Do the Bedtime Shuffle. It may seem counter-intuitive, but one of the easiest tips I have for y'all is to move up that bed time. You may have noticed that your baby has started waking earlier and earlier, right alongside the sun, even after you invested in the heavy-duty blackout curtains and white-noise machine—even springing for a fancy one that projects pictures on the ceiling. I hate to break it to you, but babies really won't be able to appreciate all those gadgets until they are at least one, but I digress.

I have found that the earlier they wake, the earlier the bedtime. My children used to sleep 9:30 to 9 like clockwork, until one day they woke up at 9, then 8, then 7, and now my toddler is poking my eyeballs at 5 a.m. every single day. Once we made their bedtime earlier at night to reflect their new morning schedule, it gave us both a break. I did have to adjust to going to bed a little earlier myself, so I could function with their bodies' natural rising time. This may be a battle for you, so feel free to use your coffee maker liberally the first week or two while you make it your new normal.

39. The Night is Dark and Full of Snoring. Well, I did mention it earlier. The blackout curtains are worth their weight in gold. You really don't need to buy the most expensive curtains, but let's be real here, a quality set of curtains can *Bill Nye Voice* Change The World. Seriously, they are life changing. If you've tried everything under the sun but this, go to the store and buy some or click on your favorite online store—just read the reviews first.

40. **Shift to the side or roll over.** Safe sleep practices tell you that back is best, and that is true. However, years ago, doctors said that babies should sleep on their stomachs, and in other countries, babies co-sleep, so it's hard to gauge what exactly is really *the* best . . . besides the one that actually gets the baby to sleep. This is why it's very important to trust your gut as a parent.

Do your research, talk to your doctor, and at the end of the day, if your baby rolls onto her tummy every single night and sleeps peacefully, that might be the way to go in your home. Some babies prefer stomach sleeping and side sleeping, but I do encourage you to wait until they are at least four months old and have strong enough neck muscles to lift their heads. But above all, talk to your doctor first.

41. Monkey See, Monkey Do. Desperate times call for desperate measures. If you're sleeping, or your baby thinks you're sleeping, they can be lulled into falling into slumber. My husband was the best at wrapping our son in a blankie on his chest and rubbing his back, until the soothing sounds of my hubby's breathing and heartbeat lulled our son to sleep. It worked almost every time, and my husband could sneak out after with minimal effort. If I were to try to move an inch away in that situation, it wouldn't work, so (bonus tip here!) try switching things up with the non-primary caregiver once in a while.

WHAT WORKED FOR YOU?

Tip	Success	Fail
Squat, baby, squat!	☐	☐
Always have a backup	☐	☐
Dancing Queen	☐	☐
Avoid eye contact	☐	☐
Heating pad	☐	☐
Heartbeat Bear	☐	☐
Bedtime Shuffle	☐	☐
Revising the Blackout	☐	☐
Side or stomach sleeping	☐	☐
Monkey See, Monkey Do	☐	☐

CHAPTER SIX
MOTION OF THE OCEAN

When you were little, you probably either fell asleep in the car . . . or you got carsick. Hopefully your baby is more favorable to the sleeping bit. Using motion as a "trick" to put babies to sleep is one of the tried-and-true methods of all generations, and luckily, we have created new ways to simulate the soothing sensation.

42. Go for a ride. It's a classic for a reason, and that reason is pretty darn simple: It works. Almost all babies will fall asleep in the car under the right circumstances. Think of your baby like your great aunt's secret brownie recipe that you need to get *just right* in order to make the ideal brownies, or else the whole thing will be ruined.

Arm yourself with white noise, a binky, his blankie, and Mom's shirt from yesterday. Or if you're lucky, take the one she was wearing before you leave the house and, like always, make sure you are awake

>>

enough to drive the vehicle and strap the baby in properly according to the car seat manual.

Whatever you do, do not leave the house without feeding the baby or bringing along milk if you plan to take a trip longer than just around the block. Just make sure to never leave your child unattended in a car seat and take the baby out of the car seat once you are back home. You don't want to leave them in the seats for too long because it raises some safety concerns, so you may only want to use this tip if you are a pro at transferring your angel to their crib.

43. Clean, clean, clean. I will keep repeating this until the end of time—or until the end of the book: babies love repetitive rocking motions. It mimics what they felt in the womb. You can suffer and hold your child until your hip hurts while you clean your house from top to bottom, or you can pop that bug in a carrier so it's a little less painful. Cleaning is a win-win, because you can finally get to those dirty socks that have been piling up in a corner and clean the toilet bowl (even though your spouse swears they did). Their clean is never as clean as your clean, and you will finally feel better afterward. Just make sure you use some family-friendly cleaners that are non-toxic and safe to use around the babe.

44. Work it Old School. Now, they may be before your time, because I know they were before mine, but for some reason, old workout videos did wonders for making my babies sleep. When they were really little, I would just walk in place, but as they got older, my kids loved to be in the carriers as I squatted and bopped around. As toddlers, they loved to copy the moves on the television with me. This is great for making them run out some of their energy and fall asleep more easily at bedtime.

45. Use the spin cycle. If you've got a dryer and you're awake enough to supervise your baby the entire time while you are actively doing laundry, saddle up for this mom hack. You can put your baby in their car seat on top of the dryer as it runs to simulate being in the car. As long as you are fully awake to monitor your baby's breathing and to make sure they're not going to fall off, you are golden. JK, who am I kidding? My kids sleep through the night now, and I'm still not awake enough to do this. I've changed my mind—don't do this. But it'd be nice, right? *Never leave your child unattended.*

46. Stroller baby: If all else fails and the weather is nice, don't be afraid to rock your unwashed hair, stained sweatshirt, and overall unhygienic postpartum mess into the outside world. A walk in the fresh air will do you both good. And if your babe is older, the new sights, smells, and sounds will distract them from crying for at least ten minutes and then they will hopefully pass out from the motion of their stroller. I like to dress my kids nice and snug with their favorite blankie, play some soothing music on speaker on my phone, and just aimlessly walk in an easy loop so when they pass out, I can park their stroller in my front yard and sit on my front stoop and connect to the Wi-Fi. #momoftheyear

WHAT WORKED FOR YOU?

Tip	Success	Fail
Go for a ride	☐	☐
Clean, clean, clean	☐	☐
Work It Old School	☐	☐
Spin cycle	☐	☐
Stroller baby	☐	☐

CHAPTER SEVEN
ROUTINE ROULETTE

The circle of life; the daily grind; same old, same old. People are creatures of habit. It makes us feel safe, in control, and secure. Life is all about routines because most humans thrive on them, and babies especially can benefit from a good schedule. It helps them know what to expect in their day-to-day, and feel comfortable that they know Mama will always feed them at eight in the morning, or Dada is going to give them a bath every night, no matter what. Comfort and security can only aid in the battle of bedtime, so here are some tips to figure out which type of schedule can work for you.

47. Eat, sleep, play, repeat: Schedules are important for babies. They might fight you at first, and it may seem like they don't want them, but they really, really do. The trick is finding the right schedule for your baby, and here's one of my favorites: Eat, Sleep, Play, Repeat. Once you get the hang of how long your babe needs to sleep at night and nap during the day, you can get in a good rhythm between their sleep schedules with feeding them and entertaining them. The important part is to follow your baby's cues. So my kids don't like to eat, sleep, play. They always eat, sleep, eat, play, eat, sleep, eat, play, eat, sleep. They are two growing boys who could literally eat all day, but hey, it worked for us.

When I first learned this tip, I thought I had to stick to it by the book, because that's what most first-time moms do. We worry, we follow everybody else's instructions, and we're too tired to know what our mom instinct is trying to tell us to do. After failing a thousand and one times, I learned to follow my babies' cues, and this tip is definitely still one of my top tools even with my toddlers. Babies and toddlers both rub their eyes when they're tired and they also fall down like they're drunk. When they're hungry, babies try to suckle and toddlers will literally try to eat you or the furniture. Just give yourself some time and you will learn how to wrangle them into a decently orderly fashion.

48. Bed = Sleep. It's a pretty simple idea, but your baby's room should be for sleep and sleep only.

Yes. Sleep, and sleep only. It can be easy to use the crib as a safe place for timeouts, or just to put your tot down for a bit while you do the dishes and clean up, but that can create some bad sleep associations.

It comes from the same mentality where adults are told not to keep televisions, music, or video games in their bedrooms because it can make it hard for them to fall asleep. The same goes for our sweet little babies. Which means that if you can afford the space, try to keep the toys in another room, or at least just keep them out of the crib.

49. Family quiet time: As I'm sure you've read before, it's important to wind down before bedtime. Take this time to set a good example by starting quiet time with the whole family, by setting aside all technology and bright lights. Bring out the books and relaxing movements to try and soothe your angel into a relaxed state.

50. Set the scene: Pretend like you're setting the scene for the most important night of your life. FYI: this is it. Your sleep is precious, so don't skimp. Pull out the Aveeno lavender-scented lotion, white noise, and blackout curtains. Anything and everything your sweet baby loves and finds comfort in to help ease the transition from being awake to sleeping is welcome here. Just pull it all out of the crib if it ends up in there with him while he drifts off.

51. Decrescendo: After setting the scene and prepping your stage, it is vital to wind down your baby before bedtime. Avoid television, iPads, or even upbeat music. This is especially important for babies as they get older and are easily overstimulated. As babies grow, they become more and more curious about the world around us because it's how they learn, and it can be very hard for them to relax. Try to dim the lights and encourage their bodies to accept the natural rhythm and call of the sandman yet again.

WHAT WORKED FOR YOU?

Tip	Success	Fail
Eat, Sleep, Play, Repeat	☐	☐
Bed = Sleep	☐	☐
Family quiet time	☐	☐
Set the scene	☐	☐
Decrescendo	☐	☐

CHAPTER EIGHT
MINI BATTLES

By now you've realized that babies are constantly changing, whether it be their interests or their basic biology, like control over their movements, voices, and potty training. In addition to those changes, there is a whole set of mini battles that can make sleep even more difficult. But it's okay! We know a few ways to work around those obstacles. We'll tackle these subjects in this chapter.

52. No nap? There will come a time in your baby's life when they will say no to their naps. At first, they will be simply resistant to the midday slumber fests, and then eventually, no matter how much elbow grease, love, cuddles, life hacks, and prayer sessions you have, they will not nap. For me, the first stage happened at one year old—which is the age where most babies drop down to one nap that is usually around

>>

two hours. If you're lucky, your toddler will keep that nap until the age of three.

Once they drop to one nap, you can schedule quiet time or a more relaxed activity for when they used to nap, until you all have completely adjusted to the new schedule. Your baby may still be cranky during that old nap period, making you want to try to get them to sleep, but as the days pass and their brains learn to process the stimulation in their big worlds, their temperament should relax as well.

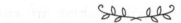

53. Germs. It's no surprise that when your baby falls ill, sleep may be hard to come by. Not only for your baby, but for you, as well. Apart from the obvious midnight wake-up calls with the NoseFrida to clean out tiny nasal passages, even when your child is fast asleep you may be too worried to shut your eyes. Trust me on this: you're no use to your babe if you do not take care of yourself, as well.

The tiny demons spreading the virus that gets past the magic of breastmilk and Lysol wipes might actually help you out with naptime and bedtime. The extra energy being used in your baby's body to fight the germs may help them fall sleep easier and sleep longer. Now, if you're not one of the lucky ones and your baby is under one year old, you may have already heard the bad news from their doctor that cold medications and the normal arsenal of pharmaceuticals that adults use are not safe for babies. Therefore, it's best to go as natural as possible for simple illnesses like the common cold.

My favorites were a hot, steamy shower to clear their congestion or, if you have the stomach of steel, the NoseFrida. If you're breastfeeding, it's best to feed your baby as much as possible because breastmilk contains antibodies that will help fight the infection and will keep your baby hydrated. By tackling these symptoms, your baby is more likely to be able to be soothed to sleep.

54. Vacation's all I ever wanted. Your routine may be perfect at home. You have your family's schedule mapped out to a tee, or you don't and your baby falls asleep the moment their angelic little bodies touch their crib . . . and then you go on vacation and everything falls apart. Little Anthony is screaming his head off and the people in the hotel room have knocked on the walls more than once because his tiny lungs produce cries louder than a baby his size should. You thought the hotel crib that they provided would be enough along with his favorite lovey, but there you are at three in the morning and Anthony is wide awake.

When you go on vacation, it's important to make the transition as smooth as possible by re-creating your baby's sleep setting as similar as possible to the cozy one you have at home. Before leaving, practice taking naps in a Pack 'n Play so you can travel with it and it isn't as unfamiliar. Bring along the sound machine you use at home, and if all else fails, you can try co-sleeping safely—no blankets, pillows, or loose clothing. You may find that even using every trick in the book, your kids may not sleep well at all, so my best advice to you is to drink a lot of coffee and pack a couple of energy drinks.

55. Milestones . . . and regressions. From the second your baby is born, they are learning new things, and with each new milestone, it may become difficult for them to sleep because their brains are learning how to take in new sensations and transition into deeper sleep cycles. This can be a stressful time for everyone, so it's very important to remember the most essential rule of parenting—you cannot take care of your baby unless you take care of yourself first.

And unfortunately, with mental leaps, there are no specific tricks that will help you get through this tough bit of time. You just have to be patient and try to not lose your minds while your babes shriek like crazy banshees even though you have tried every single thing they usually like. The good news is that this is only a temporary period, and once they get used to their new skills and aren't as overwhelmed, they will become more even tempered and should fall asleep just as easily as they did before.

56. New siblings: Big changes in the household can disrupt the sleep patterns of the most easy-going child. When it comes time to bring home a new little bundle of joy, it's important to keep your first-born's routine as similar as possible. They may not even have trouble falling asleep if you're lucky, but if you aren't, you may want to try sticking as close to your old routine as possible.

One thing about kids is that, whether they know it or not, they crave consistency and hate change. So, when you add an entirely new human being into the mix that cries every few minutes and steals Mommy's snuggles or Daddy's attention . . . well, you can be sure to add another 2 a.m. wake-up call to your list. Remember that sleep regressions are normal, temper tantrums are normal, and above all, just try and be patient and don't be afraid to call in reinforcements.

57. Oh, potty training. . . . Now this may not become an issue for a while, but some children can start potty training at an early age. This can lead to middle of the night wake-up calls to use the potty or cries to change their sheets. And as we all know, children thrive on routine. So it's important to try to fit potty training as seamlessly into their normal schedule as possible. Try getting them to go every hour, after meals, or set a repeating alarm on your phone. Find a system that works for your family, so when it comes time to sleep, their bladders are less likely to be full and in need of a middle-of-the-night potty break. It is also good to remember that wearing diapers for nighttime is completely okay until your little one is ready to wake up on their own. You may find that they sleep longer that way.

CHAPTER NINE
OLD WIVES' TALES

Old Wives' Tales—everyone knows at least one. Before you skeptically throw those ideas out the window, try to remember that babies are not allowed to have cold medicine, sleep with blankets, and do a lot of the things that actually make it easier for older children and adults to sleep when they are uncomfortable. Old wives' tales exist for a reason, and if they're harmless, why not give them a shot?

58. Perform some gymnastics: I've heard it said that when babies get gassy, a little gymnastics is all they need. The older generation suggests gently holding a gassy baby and slowly flipping them in the air while supporting their body and neck. The motions must be slow, feet over head, and at least three times to help move the trapped gas and settle the baby's stomach. This may or may not help settle your baby down for a nap, but at the very least it should ease the tension of any crying (the baby's or yours).

59. Extensions? Do they really work? Many people believe that if you keep a baby awake longer during the day, they are more likely to sleep at night. This advice can be taken wrong—please let your baby nap during the day!—but it does hold some merit, especially if you're gradually trying to switch a baby's sleep schedule around because they tend to be a night owl. The idea is that you will tire them out by keeping them awake for longer periods, thus making them want to sleep at night. Sadly, most babies can just end up overtired, cranky, and more difficult to put down. Try this old wives' tale at your own risk.

60. Sunrise, sunset. The sun is there for a reason. Try to keep it as a guide for your little babe, to help teach them that when it is light out, it's time to play, and when the sun goes down, it's time to get ready for bed. Back in the day, before we had electricity, that's what folks did and it worked for them.

61. Add some cozy socks. Babies are so tiny and helpless, and something about being an older woman makes almost all grandmothers believe that they need socks, especially at night. Many will swear that if a baby's feet are cold then they will not go to sleep. So, even if you think little Susie is snug as a bug in her fleece onesie, try putting on a pair of cotton socks underneath to see if cold feet may be keeping her up.

62. Tea time! Once your baby is on solids at six months old, most doctors say it's safe for babies to have the occasional ounce or two of herbal tea. My grandmother and countless others swear by giving babies chamomile tea. It's supposed to help calm and relax them just like it does for adults, and if your doctor gives you the green light, why not, right?

WHAT WORKED FOR YOU?

Tip	Success	Fail
Gymnastics	☐	☐
Extensions	☐	☐
Sunrise, sunset	☐	☐
Tea time	☐	☐

CHAPTER TEN
CRUNCHY MAMA

If you haven't heard of the term *crunchy moms,* you probably haven't joined a Facebook mom group. Crunchy moms take a more holistic approach to parenting, and they tend to be looked at as the hippies in the modern-day mom group. With all the warnings about toxicity of toys, bottles, and cleaners, most parents you meet will have at least given a few thoughts into making more "crunchy" parenting choices. These tips are perfect for newborns to six-month-olds, because they embrace a more natural approach to bedtime.

63. Maybe try co-sleeping. In the Western world, it is advised that parents do not co-sleep with their children for safety reasons. But every family is different, and in Eastern countries, it has been shown that

>>

bed-sharing is completely safe and beneficial to the baby as long as certain safety precautions are taken. No pillows, sheets, blankets, or stuffed animals are allowed in the bed while you are co-sleeping. The mother must not drink, smoke, or take medications. To be absolutely safe, the other partner should not be in the bed and the mother should have her hair tied back and be wearing tight-fitted clothing. If done properly, co-sleeping can have a lot of benefits.

64. Breastfeeding . . . again: It fixes everything, dontcha know? Crunchy moms everywhere swear that just boobin' it can help a baby sleep, get rid of colds, earaches, the works. And, if you are breastfeeding, it's worth a shot. Often times, babies will fall asleep breastfeeding because they can eat and sleep simultaneously—it's gotta be some sort of boob magic. Getting them off the boob and into their crib is the real problem.

If you're not okay with co-sleeping, I suggest nursing while lying on a bed, and when your babe is in a deep slumber, channel your inner ninja. Unlatch and then roll without making the mattress move too much. Then and only then can you gently scoop up your baby and softly place them in their safe sleeping space.

65. Essential oils anyone? Some mamas swear that diffusing lavender essential oils in their baby's room made their four-month-old sleep through the night. However, it's important to note that essential oils should *never* be used on a baby younger than three months, and you should always consult with a doctor. If your doc gives you the go-ahead, it is surely worth a shot; the pleasant and calming smell may be enough to help soothe your baby to sleep once in a while.

66. Wear all the babies! Or so say all the crunchy mamas in all the land. If you wear your babes and breastfeed, you are golden. All you have to do is throw in a heavy dose of essential oils and you'll be set. Whether they're in a wrap, sling, or structured carrier, the body heat from your skin, movement from walking around, and soothing sound of your heartbeat will help your babe fall asleep. Sometimes it can take a bit for your child to get used to the sensation of being in a carrier, but once you're past that hump, it's a lifesaver. You can baby-wear doing chores, on walks, and even while working out. Just make sure that the baby's airway is clear at all times and that their head is at a kissable distance.

67. Amber teething necklaces. There is no definitive evidence that the amber teething necklace works, but I have to say that, personally, I think it helps with the pain, or at least with the fussiness. My children wore their necklaces during the day when I had eyes on them, but during naps and at night I always removed them. The pain-relieving effect happens as the heat from their bodies warms the amber beads and a small amount of oil that contains succinic acid theoretically seeps into their skin. My thoughts were that if they were in less pain during the day without medication, they would sleep better at night . . . and they did. As always, follow safe sleep recommendations, *don't* allow your child to sleep in any necklace, and ask your doctor.

68. What stress? Babies have an almost sixth sense for stress, especially when it comes to their mamas. They can pick it up in the air, off your skin, from your sweat glands, and it can stress them out, too, preventing them from relaxing enough to sleep. Do yourself a favor, and if you find yourself getting too stressed from trying to put the baby down for the night, swap shifts with your partner. Even if it's just a few minutes so you can take a breather and relax, the moment to yourself will do you and baby good.

69. Be consistent: Babies thrive on routine; there are certain infants that depend on routine like their lives will end if you deviate from schedule by a minute. The cliché about being home for naptime or needing to leave early to get little Jimmy to bed on time is very, very true for some kids. Try to be courteous of this fact, and if Jimmy needs his bedtime at eight sharp, hire a babysitter or ask Grandma to come help instead of staying out later at a get-together. It will just end up making you both cranky when you're up a thousand times later that night. Okay, who am I kidding? When you're still up at 1 a.m. that night because Jim Jim is overtired now.

70. The Focker Method: If you've ever watched *Meet the Fockers*, Gaylord's parents were a little overbearing and very, very affectionate. Well, some babies thrive on that type of attention. They need to be held almost 24/7 whether you're peeing, eating, taking a step into another room—or even thinking about doing so. With this method, you will basically coddle your child to sleep and answer every cry immediately, with 100 percent effort every time, because if they feel secure enough in your love, they should feel secure enough to sleep.

71. Body odor: Biology is freakin' weird, and babies love the way their mamas smell. Smelling their mama close by is one of the most relaxing things in the entire world for a new little baby. To help trick your babe into thinking you're nearby, try wearing their crib sheet all day while you're in the house and put it on their bed before you put them to sleep for the night. The smell that you leave behind can help get you some extra ZZZs.

WHAT WORKED FOR YOU?

Tip	Success	Fail
Co-sleeping	☐	☐
Breastfeeding to sleep	☐	☐
Essential oils	☐	☐
Wear all the babies!	☐	☐
Amber teething necklace	☐	☐
Manage your stress	☐	☐
Be consistent	☐	☐
The Focker Method	☐	☐
Body odor	☐	☐

CHAPTER ELEVEN
BIOLOGICAL WARFARE

It happens to us all—we get sick and our bodies don't allow us to sleep. Back in the good ol' days that we daydream about, we used to sleep until noon on the weekends, or if we're lucky, on a sick day. We could binge-watch Netflix without a care in the world and take NyQuil without worrying about needing to stay alert to change a diaper. Now, having a sick baby is a whole other story! Babies have a tougher time than adults because they can't use most "good" medicines that make people comfortable enough to sleep. Our little angels are uncomfortable and cranky, which can affect their sleep, but luckily there are a few tricks to make the sniffles less awful.

72. Suck it up! If you haven't heard, there is this semi-magical device that allows you to suck snot out of your child's nose. It's called the NoseFrida. It is one of the best and worst things ever created. If you have a weak stomach, I recommend getting your partner to do it, but trust me, it helps. This baby will clear out those nasal cavities like no other nose sucker out there, and at the very least a congested nose will not keep your baby awake.

73. Hook up a humidifier. If your baby has a stuffy nose from the common cold, a humidifier can do wonders in making them more comfortable during naptime or bedtime. Make sure to add it to your baby registry, so when baby's first cold rolls around, you can be prepared and make a restless night a little easier!

74. Steamy weather. Now, if your humidifier is on the fritz or you're unable to buy one, you can use this tried-and-true method of a hot steamy shower. It works great for steaming wrinkles out of your favorite fancy outfit as well as clearing up little Ben's nasal passages. Bring a few toys in to help distract your child from having to stay in the bathroom for a while or simply rock them while the steam works its magic. Being able to breathe easier will make putting him to sleep a lot easier on both of you.

75. Q-Tip magic. This one is kind of weird, even for me. Gas is a normal human function for all people, but teeny babies can have a very difficult time pushing out toots. If this happens, it can make it beyond difficult for them to sleep. Take a q-tip and put a liberal amount of Vaseline on the tip. Gently and very carefully push it in your baby's bum just as if you were to take their temperature. The stimulation of the q-tip can help get gas moving and alleviate some of the discomfort. If you are feeling fancy and want to keep things more twenty-first century, you can buy a Baby Windi, which also helps relieve gas and colic like a q-tip. Personally, my doctor told me about the q-tip so that was our go-to, but you can ask yours what they think is best!

76. Create a fart machine. If your baby is still gassy after a little q-tip trick, gripe water can be a huge life-saver. It can help release the trapped gas bubbles in your baby's tummy. If gripe water does not work, you can try the gas drop simethicone. Ask your doctor first, of course, and then follow the directions on the box.

77. And . . . more farts. Yes, I'm still talking about gas here. Another great lifesaver is a gentle tummy massage with some coconut oil to get things moving. There are even YouTube videos that show you various techniques, but my all-time favorite is simply placing my hands around my baby's tummy, so my thumbs are on his belly and my fingers are on his back, and then gently squeezing and sliding my fingers toward his lower belly like I'm squeezing the most fragile toothpaste container in the world. Be prepared for a blowout diaper, because all these tips combined will definitely get rid of any gas problems preventing your baby from sleeping.

78. All about the angles! Math class can actually come in handy now that you have kids. It turns out that something as simple as a baby sleeping at a slight angle can help soothe acid reflux and some-times even gas. It can be as simple as putting a folded towel under one part of the mattress and between the crib springs, so one side of the bed is slightly elevated. When your baby lies down with their head on the higher end, the acid is less likely to hurt them. This was one of the tricks we learned when my youngest had extremely bad acid reflux, and medication still barely helped. Please first talk to your doctor about the safety and whether this tip will be safe and help-ful for your child.

79. Put some rice cereal in the bottle. The rice cereal debate about making babies sleep longer is mostly a myth, *but* it does stem from some truth. If a baby has acid reflux, adding a touch of rice cereal can help reduce the pain they experience from reflux, which may help them sleep longer. Talk to your doctor about possible reflux and a rice-to-breastmilk or formula ratio. It is a very, very small amount.

80. Consider medication. If your baby is up screaming and is completely inconsolable no matter what you do, it's time to call your doctor. They may be teething, have an ear infection, or could be experiencing acid reflux and need medication to help. A doctor can help you decide the best course of treatment and get your baby on the best medication to help, if it's necessary. Modern medicine is a wonderful thing, and once you treat the root of the problem and your baby is no longer uncomfortable from being sick or teething, they should return to their normal sleep routine.

WHAT WORKED FOR YOU?

Tip	Success	Fail
NoseFrida	☐	☐
Humidifier	☐	☐
Steam	☐	☐
Q-Tip magic	☐	☐
Fart machine	☐	☐
Tummy massage	☐	☐
Angles	☐	☐
Rice cereal	☐	☐
Medications	☐	☐

CHAPTER TWELVE
PLAYING HARDBALL

Okay, enough is enough. You've been getting up every hour for maybe eight or nine months now and this morning you tried to feed your cat a bottle. It's time to sleep-train. I know some parents disagree with sleep-training and may call it a little harsh. Taking this step can be very hard. With your hormones still regulating postpartum, or if you have a very sympathetic personality, you may find it nearly impossible to let your baby cry when you can almost hear other moms judging your parenting decisions.

It's okay. Take a deep breath. Sleep-training is a perfectly acceptable, and safe, choice for families. If you are concerned, talk to your doctor, but don't let the fear and stigma from Facebook mom groups stop you from doing what is right for your family. For me, I personally loved sleep-training for my family. I am a very, very, hands-on parent who is all for attachment parenting, but it got to a point where nothing else worked and my eldest needed a firmer hand at night to fall asleep. Sometimes, you have to give a little tough love in order to take care of yourself and your baby.

Remember, if you're not sleeping and your baby is not sleeping, it's not healthy for either of you. These tips will help you sleep-train in a gentle way if you choose, so it's easier on both of you.

81. The Ferber Method. The Ferber Method was created by Dr. Ferber because he believed that the most efficient way to teach a child to sleep was to allow them to cry at bedtime. Hence the term *cry it out*. Now, before you get too excited, it's not as bad as it first sounds. The baby needs to be *at least* six months old and preferably not eating during the middle of the night, and as always, talk to your doctor first.

This method relies on having a strict routine and putting your baby to sleep in their own room. Dr. Ferber recommends checking in on your baby at intervals. First after three minutes, five minutes, and ten minutes on the first day. Then on the second day, the intervals increase to five, ten, and twelve. On the third day to ten minutes and eventually twenty minutes on day seven.

During each check on your baby, you should soothe them *without* picking them up. You can pat their back, shush them, and then leave the room right before she falls asleep. Your baby should start self-soothing and learn to fall asleep by herself around day five, and if it doesn't work after the first try, you may just need to try it a few weeks later, because every baby is different (Ferber, 2016).

82. The Jodi Mindell Method. Dr. Jodi A. Mindell's first bit of advice is for parents to chill the F out about their baby's sleep habits—especially new parents. After twelve weeks, she recommends a consistent routine, an early bedtime, and letting your baby self-soothe. Which, to Mindell, means do not jump out of bed at your little angel's first whimper, but give them a few minutes to work it out themselves (Mindell, 1997).

83.   The Baby Wise Method. Baby Wise promotes an Eat-Play-Sleep schedule, where your child wakes up, feeds, and engages in an activity before ultimately going down for a nap. The goal is for parents to put their baby down in their cribs drowsy but awake. They recommend around two hours between feedings for newborns, three hours after the first couple of months, and eventually four hours. They believe that spreading out feedings can encourage babies to sleep through the night by four months old since they are eating more at one time (Bucknam & Ezzo, 2015).

84. The Baby Whisperer Method. The Baby Whisperer is very similar to Baby Wise, but instead implements an ever so slightly altered routine: E.A.S.Y. This stands for Eat, Activity, Sleep, and You Time. Surface level, it's like Baby Wise, but the creator, Tracy Hogg, makes it very clear that it's is a literal *easy* routine that is not meant to be strict, and it's okay for one day to look different from another. This method is more clock-based and about following your baby's lead, encouraging your child into better sleep habits. Hogg also makes it very clear that parents need to watch for their baby's cues in order for this method to work (Hogg, 2005).

85. The Weissbluth Method. If you have a problem with cry it out, this is not the method for you, so skip to Tip 86. Still here? Okay, so, the Weissbluth method uses extinction, a.k.a. no comfort to stop your baby from crying at night. Weissbluth instructs parents to put their babies down to sleep and not to go into their room unless there is an emergency. It is also recommended to have shorter and fewer naps during the day to help your baby sleep better at night. This method should never be used on a child younger than six months, or before talking to their pediatrician. Some experts do say that this could teach your baby learned helplessness, while others say that by using the method properly and watching your baby's cues, it can help them learn to self-soothe faster than the Ferber Method (Weissbluth, 2015).

86. The No-Cry Sleep Method. Now, if you've made it through all of these sleep-training options, and none feel right for your family, this may be more your style. *The No-Cry Sleep Solution* by Elizabeth Pantley encourages parents to rock and feed their babies until they get drowsy and then put them down. If the baby cries, she says to respond immediately. She also urges parents to log lengths of naps, sleep at night, and night-wakings (Pantley, 2002). I think of it as Diet Sleep Training because you are still not putting your babe down when they are completely asleep. It helps them learn how to transition on their own but with a very supportive presence of their parent.

WHAT WORKED FOR YOU?

Tip	Success	Fail
The Ferber Method	☐	☐
The Jody Mindell Method	☐	☐
The Baby Wise Method	☐	☐
The Baby Whisperer Method	☐	☐
The Weissbluth Method	☐	☐
The No-Cry Sleep Method	☐	☐

CHAPTER THIRTEEN
PARENTING ARMOR

The first year of parenting a baby is one of the toughest. A lot of moms go through postpartum depression, and even some dads experience some type of depression, as well. Taking care of a tiny human, being their sole source of comfort, food, and safety is a taxing experience even on the strongest of us. It's okay to be stressed out. It's okay to need space. It's okay to cry in the bathroom.

You *will* survive this time period. If you find yourself coping in an unhealthy way, you need to reach out to someone—a doctor, friend, family member. Just someone. Therefore, it's VERY important for you to take care of yourself before you have a full-on meltdown from lack of sleep, stress, or postpartum depression. At the very least, you need to take some time to yourself. Hire a babysitter, call up Grandma, or just take a bubble bath while eating some chocolate after your baby finally goes to sleep. Until then, here are some tips to help you get through the battle.

87. Plug 'em up! You can do everything possible and your baby can still scream. Many refer to the evening hours before bedtime as *the witching hour*, after all. Despite every trick in the book, your baby may still scream. But if they're not in pain, they don't have a fever, and they're acting healthy otherwise, then try not to feel guilty when you reach for the earplugs. Invest in a good pair of earplugs or headphones so you can rock the baby and bounce around the house for hours without your ears bleeding during the day.

88. Find a good distraction. Audio books, music, YouTube, memes—one or more of these will become your best friends while you're rocking your baby to sleep at night. Midnight feeds while rocking your sweet angel in their recliner will become a precarious exercise of wills as you try not to fall asleep holding your precious bundle of joy. Distractions will also help keep you sane when your child won't stop crying no matter what you do. Reminder: adorable cat memes will do wonders to lighten the mood when your ears are about to bleed from the surprisingly loud wails from their tiny lungs.

89. Spend some quality time. Date night with your partner, intimacy, time alone. Anything and everything that makes you two connect over more than the color of your baby's poop. If you can't afford or trust anyone to babysit, down an energy drink or a cup of coffee after the baby goes to bed one night a month and just hang out with your partner. And if you're up to it, get lucky—it will make you both feel so much better.

90. Call in the reinforcements! Repeat after me: "It's okay to ask for help." Okay, now say it again and again until you stop feeling guilty. Okay, joking. That will never happen, but maybe it will take the edge off. It's totally okay to pick up the phone and call in Grandma or Grandpa to take over a few night shifts once in a while so you can catch up on sleep. Especially if you're the mama. After all, you just created life and your body is still recovering from that experience.

WHAT WORKED FOR YOU?

Tip	Success	Fail
Ear plugs	☐	☐
Distractions	☐	☐
Quality time	☐	☐
Reinforcements	☐	☐

CHAPTER FOURTEEN
BOUNDARIES

When you first get pregnant, you may be super against bed-sharing, but then that's the only way your baby will fall asleep. Or you hate how your baby pulls your hair, but again, it's the only way they fall asleep. Days, then weeks, and then months pass, and then you finally realize that the sleep you're getting isn't good enough. Or the pain you're receiving is too much and you can't deal with it. You snap at your spouse, you snap at your dog, and you might even yell at your baby.

At one point, you will explode. Or you will almost explode and want to just scream, cry, or hit something. ALWAYS remember that it's okay to put your baby down in a safe spot, like their crib or their nursery if it is baby-proofed, so you can take a few minutes to calm down. This is not the same as Cry It Out—it simply is a way to keep everyone safe until you can function again.

The goal, however, is to avoid getting to that point, and to do that, you need to set boundaries. I know, I know—you're a parent, and their adorable chubby cheeks and annoying squealing cries are hard to say no to, but your health is vital for the health or your family—remember that.

91. My nips, not your nips. If you breastfed for any length of time, your baby may be slightly obsessed with your nipples. You may have weaned and they still want to twiddle for comfort, or they like holding on to the opposite nipple as they nurse. Now, it may seem cute at first, but baby and toddler nails can be wicked sharp and can do some damage as they are trying to soothe themselves to sleep. Don't be afraid to tell them no for your own sanity, wear a sports bra, or at the very least put long socks on their hands as you rock them to sleep so they can find another source of comfort that does not chip away at you mentally and cause extra stress.

92. The marriage bed woes. This is a large source of contention between many, many couples, because despite making promises to ourselves and each other, some of us inevitably end up with a baby or toddler in our bed at night. It makes things simpler most of the time, but undoubtedly one partner will be less than thrilled when they turn over to snuggle their partner and get a stinky toddler foot to the face. Or worse—feel the horror of a leaky diaper on their pillow. So that's when they draw the line. No more co-sleeping in their bed.

Which is fine. There are many solutions, including making your partner the Manager in Charge of middle of the night wake-up calls. After a week or two of little Johnny refusing to go back to sleep, they may not complain anymore. Or if this is the final call for you both, it's time to do what I like to call Co-Sleep Weaning. You can do it cold turkey, or you can gradually try to move into this transition with a PJ Masks bedding set and stuffed animal bribe to motivate your child. You know your child best, so try to remember that every transition will be hard, but the boundaries you set for your mental health will only benefit them in the long run.

93. Last call for boob milk! Whether you wanted to breastfeed for a week, six months, or three years, you ultimately need to remember that your breasts are a part of *your* body. Yes, breastfeeding has amazing benefits for mom and baby, but if at any time you're feeling run down, angry, or even touched out for every single feeding, it's time to put up some boundaries with breastfeeding even if it's the only way your child will go to sleep easily. There are dozens of ways you can help your baby get used to falling asleep without the boob, and if you're not feeling happy while breastfeeding, eventually that stress will be passed along to your child and can make it difficult for them to fall asleep anyway.

ACHIEVEMENT UNLOCKED

If you read the whole book without putting yourself to sleep first, then you definitely need to cut back on your caffeine intake. I know putting your baby to bed is difficult, but if you're loaded up with five-hour energy, you're not going to sleep well either. I hope these tips and tricks can make putting your sweet little baby to sleep just a wee bit easier than soothing a stray cat. Good luck and godspeed, because once your child sleeps through the night, new challenges will begin!

ACHIEVEMENT
UNLOCKED

ABOUT THE AUTHOR

Melissa Guida-Richards is an author and stay-at-home mother to two beautiful boys. She has a bachelor of arts degree in psychology and criminal justice that helped her hone her research skills, which has become essential to her success as a millennial mama. Her blog, Spoonie-Mama, chronicles her experiences as a toddler mama with chronic pain, mental illness, and her journey of self-discovery as an adoptee. You can find her writing on *Zora by Medium*, *The Huffington Post*, *Motherly*, *Her View From Home*, *Filter Free Parents*, *Scary Mommy*, and more. You can check out more of her writing at Guida-Richards.com.

She gave birth to her first child in 2016, and it's safe to say a good night's sleep was a distant memory after that. It took six months to get her first child to sleep through the night, and eight months with her youngest. She searched everywhere to find the trick to getting her babies a good night's rest; digging deep into online forums, mom blogs, nanny chats, old wives' tales, and Facebook mom groups. Each piece of advice helped . . . until it didn't. Until teething, sleep regressions, or growth spurts. Then it was a whole new ball game trying to get her once happy napper to go down during the day, just as he did at night. So, once again, she took to the Internet for answers.

It took dozens of tries to find the answer for her family, and she suspected that there wasn't one. When her second child was born in 2017, she learned the disappointing truth: it doesn't get easier with the second baby. There is a learning curve where the parent and child must take time to learn how to help one another. It was hard, and many times she almost gave up, until she realized that she had the answers at her fingertips. She just needed to start from the top and test *all* the methods to get a baby to sleep until she found the one that worked best.

REFERENCES

Bucknam, Robert MD. and Gary Ezzo. *ON BECOMING BABY WISE: Giving Your Infant the Gift of Nighttime Sleep* (Parent-Wise Solutions, Inc. 2015) ISBN-10: 1932740139.

Ferber, Richards MD. *Solve Your Child's Sleep Problems.* (Touchstone, 2006) ISBN-10: 0743201639.

Hogg, Tracy. *The Baby Whisperer Solves All Your Problems (by Teaching You How to Ask the Right Questions)* (Vermilion, 2005) ISBN-10: 0091902517.

Mindell, Jodi A. *Sleeping Through the Night: How Infants, Toddlers, And Their Parents Can Get A Good Night's Sleep.* (Collins, 1997) ISBN-10: 0062734091.

Pantley, Elizabeth. *The No-Cry Sleep Solution: Gentle Ways to Help Your Baby Sleep Through the Night* (McGraw-Hill Education, 2002) ISBN-10: 0071381392.

Weissbluth, Marc MD. *Healthy Sleep Habits, Happy Child, 4th Edition: A Step-by-Step Program for a Good Night's Sleep* (Ballantine Books 2015) ISBN-10: 0553394800.

REFERENCES

ACKNOWLEDGMENTS

To my husband, Charles Richards II, and my two sons, Carlito and Killian . . . I could not have written this book without you. Every late night we had together helped shape all of the tips in this book. I love you more than you can ever know.

I have to thank my awesome critique partner, Danielle Renino. She has been with me on this writing journey every step of the way. Danielle read my early drafts, blurbs, and pieces of my proposal without complaint. Thank you so much for being a great friend.

A million thanks to my early readers: Mackenzie Eyler, my mom Paula Guida, and my dear friend Athena Otten. You helped give me valuable insight on what worked and what didn't. I would also like to thank my editor, Nicole Frail, for her help making this book what it is. She has been so kind and helpful throughout this whole process.

I would also like to thank my mom and dad, Rocco Guida, for coming around and supporting my new passion. It meant a lot every time you would talk about my book and ask how many words I wrote that day. Last, but not least, I would like to thank my dear friends Alissa Jolley, Alex Lefever, and Samantha Krushinsky for being there for me. Your emotional support meant more than you know.

INDEX

NOTES

....

....

....

....

....

....

....

....

....

....

....

....

....

....

....

....

··

··

··

··

··

··

··

··

··

··

··

··

··

··

··

··

....

....

....

....

....

....

....

....

....

....

....

....

....

....

....

....

....

....

....

....

....

....

....

....

....

....

....

....

....

....

....